AFFIRMATION STUDIOS

101 AFFIRMATIONS FOR ANXIETY

Positive Affirmations for an Abundant Life

AFFIRMATION STUDIOS

101 Affirmations for Anxiety

Positive Affirmations for an Abundant Life

Contents

Welcome

Here at Affirmation Studio, we want to provide the power of affirmations so that you have the ability to become who you want to be.

The next two chapters will go over Anxiety and Affirmations. If you would like to jump straight to the affirmations, please go to chapter 3, 101 Anxiety Affirmations.

We included each affirmation on its own page for your convenience, to make personal notes, tear out your favorite pages to keep them with you, or even proudly display them on your walls as a constant reminder of positivity and abundance!

Now let's dive in.

Chapter 1: Anxiety

What is Anxiety?

Anxiety is a feeling of worry, nervousness, or unease about something with an uncertain outcome. It is a normal and often healthy emotion, but it can become overwhelming or chronic when it interferes with daily activities. Anxiety disorders are one of the most common mental disorders in the world and affect millions of people.

Symptoms of anxiety can include:
- Restlessness
- A feeling of being wound up or on edge
- Irritability
- Muscle Tension
- Difficulty Concentrating
- Sleep Disturbances
- Physical Symptoms
    - Rapid Heartbeat
    - Sweating

The exact causes of anxiety are not fully understood but may involve a combination of genetic, environmental, and lifestyle factors.

Anxiety & Affirmations

Positive affirmations are statements or phrases designed to counteract negative thoughts and promote self-confidence and well-being. They can play a role in managing anxiety by helping to reframe negative and self-critical thoughts and replace them with more positive and empowering beliefs.

The repetitive and consistent use of positive affirmations can help to retrain the brain to focus on the present moment and recognize negative thought patterns. This can help to reduce feelings of anxiety and promote a sense of calm and stability. Positive affirmations can also boost self-esteem and help counteract the effects of anxiety-provoking thoughts, allowing the person to feel more in control of their emotions and reactions.

It's important to note that while positive affirmations can be a helpful tool for managing anxiety, they should not be used as a replacement for professional treatment. For some individuals, anxiety may require medication, therapy, or a combination of both for effective management.

Chapter 2: Affirmations

What are Affirmations?

Affirmations are positive statements or declarations that are used to challenge and overcome negative thoughts, beliefs, and emotions. The goal of affirmations is to replace negative self-talk with positive, empowering messages that support and encourage personal growth, self-esteem, and well-being. Affirmations can be used to focus on specific areas of life, such as relationships, careers, health, or finances. They can also be general statements promoting positive thinking and outlook on life. When used regularly, affirmations can help to change limiting beliefs and create a more positive mindset, leading to increased happiness, confidence, and overall well-being.

Do Affirmations Actually Work?

Affirmations can be a helpful tool for many people, but it's important to remember that they are not a magic solution and may only work for some. However, there is scientific evidence to support the benefits of using affirmations.

Studies have shown that repeating affirmations can change how we think and feel about ourselves and the world around us. Affirmations can help reduce stress and anxiety, improve mood, and increase self-esteem and overall well-being. They can also help boost motivation and productivity and foster a growth mindset, which is essential for personal and professional growth.

However, the effectiveness of affirmations depends on several factors, including the type of affirmations used, how often they are repeated, and the individual's level of belief and commitment to the affirmations. It's also essential to choose affirmations that resonate with you and to repeat them regularly, which will help to train your brain to focus on positive thoughts and beliefs.

While affirmations may not work for everyone, they can be a powerful tool for personal growth and improvement when used correctly. It's always a good idea to consult with a mental health professional if you are struggling with anxiety or other mental health issues to determine the best course of action.

How do Affirmations Work?

Our thoughts and beliefs shape our reality, so negative thoughts and beliefs can lead to negative experiences and emotions. Affirmations provide a powerful tool to help counteract this cycle by introducing positive thoughts and beliefs into our consciousness. Affirmations work by rewiring the brain and changing negative thought patterns into positive ones.

The repetitive nature of affirmations is vital for their effectiveness. By repeating affirmations regularly, we can train our brain to focus on positive thoughts and beliefs and change how we think about ourselves and the world around us. Over time, this can lead to a shift in our mindset, increasing our self-esteem and overall well-being.

Moreover, when we make an affirmation, we are making a declaration of intent, and this intentional declaration has a profound impact on our subconscious mind. Our subconscious mind doesn't discriminate between what's real and imagined, so when we repeat affirmations, our subconscious mind begins to believe them. This belief drives our thoughts, behaviors, and emotions.

In summary, affirmations work by introducing positive thoughts and beliefs into our consciousness, repetition trains the brain to focus on these positive thoughts, and the declaration of intent profoundly impacts the subconscious mind, leading to lasting change.

Chapter 3: 101 Anxiety Affirmations

1. I am calm and in control.
2. I trust in my ability to handle any situation.
3. I am safe and protected.
4. I choose peace and let go of worry.
5. I am strong and capable.
6. I am surrounded by love and support.
7. I am worthy and deserving of happiness.
8. I am courageous.
9. I release all fear and embrace positivity.
10. I am capable of managing my anxiety.
11. I am grateful for this moment and all that I have.
12. I am enough exactly as I am.
13. I am worthy of love and respect.
14. I am able to overcome any challenge.
15. I am filled with inner peace and calm.
16. I choose to focus on the present moment.
17. I am surrounded by positive energy.
18. I am worthy.
19. I am capable of handling anything that comes my way.
20. I am grateful for my life and all its blessings.
21. I trust the journey of life.

22. I choose to let go of negative thoughts.

23. I am strong and resilient.

24. I am worthy of a life filled with joy.

25. I am confident.

26. I am at peace with where I am in life.

27. I am worthy of a life filled with fulfillment and purpose.

28. I am in control of my mind.

29. I am capable of overcoming any obstacle.

30. I am deserving of a life filled with peace and happiness.

31. I am surrounded by positive people who support me.

32. I am worthy of success and prosperity.

33. I am at peace with myself and the world around me.

34. I have a happy and fulfilling life.

35. I choose to focus on the good in every situation.

36. I choose to live each day with joy and positivity.

37. I am worthy of a life filled with success.

38. I am surrounded by positive, supportive people.

39. I am at peace with the present moment.

40. I am deserving of a life filled with love and fulfillment.

41. I choose to focus on my goals and aspirations.

42. I am capable of finding solutions to any problem.

43. I am at peace with the journey of life.

44. I am grateful for my many blessings.

45. I am in control of my thoughts and emotions.

46. I am surrounded by positive energy and love.

47. I am grateful for the present moment and all that it brings.

48. I am worthy of an abundant life.

49. I am able to find joy and happiness in every situation.

50. I trust in my own abilities and decisions.

51. I am deserving of a life filled with love, peace, and happiness.

52. I am strong and accomplished.

53. I am grateful for my journey and all that I have learned.

54. I am capable of managing my thoughts and emotions.

55. I am in control of my reactions to stressful situations.

56. I am strong and capable of facing any challenge.

57. I am worthy of love, peace, and happiness.

58. I am deserving of a life filled with success and abundance.

59. I focus on my own progress, not perfection.

60. I am surrounded by a supportive network of friends and family.

61. I am grateful for the opportunities life presents to me.

62. I am deserving of a life filled with love and positivity.

63. I am strong and capable of overcoming any barrier.

64. I am at peace with my past and excited for my future.

65. I am deserving of a fulfilling and meaningful life.

66. I focus on the present and let go of worries.

67. I am worthy of love and happiness in all areas of my life.

68. I am capable of finding joy in even the most difficult situations.

69. I am surrounded by positive energy and positivity.

70. I am deserving of success and abundance in all areas of my life.

71. I am capable of facing any challenge.

72. I am grateful for my health and well-being.

73. I am calm and centered in every moment.

74. I am without worry.

75. I am capable of handling any situation with ease.

76. I am overcoming anxiety.

77. I am surrounded by love and positivity.

78. I am strong and resilient in the face of stress.

79. I am letting go of the past and future.

80. I am worthy of love and happiness.

81. I trust my life's journey.

82. I am fearless.

83. I am enough just as I am.

84. I am surrounded by abundance and prosperity.

85. I am confident in my decisions and trust my intuition.

86. I am worthy of a life free from anxiety.

87. I am grateful for the peace and serenity in my life.

88. I am capable of achieving my goals and dreams.

89. I am strong and capable of handling anything that comes my way.

90. I am at peace with the uncertainty of life.

91. I am filled with love and positivity.

92. I am joyful and peaceful.

93. I am free from worry and stress.

94. I am graceful and resilient.

95. I am deserving of a life filled with happiness and success.

96. I am surrounded by a supportive network of people who love and care for me.

97. I am grateful for my life.

98. I am valid in my feelings.

99. I am under no threat from the world.

100. I am calmer and more relaxed with each new day.

101. I am in control of my life.

I am calm and in control.

I trust in my ability to handle any situation.

I am safe and protected.

I choose peace and let
go of worry.

I am strong and
capable.

I am surrounded by love
and support.

I am worthy and deserving of happiness.

I am courageous.

I release all fear and embrace positivity.

I am capable of

managing my anxiety.

I am grateful for this
moment and all that I
have.

I am enough exactly as I am.

I am worthy of love and

respect.

I am able to overcome

any challenge.

I am filled with inner
peace and calm.

I choose to focus on the
present moment.

I am surrounded by

positive energy.

I am worthy.

I am capable of
handling anything that
comes my way.

I am grateful for my life
and all its blessings.

I trust the journey of life.

I choose to let go of

negative thoughts.

I am strong and
resilient.

I am worthy of a life

filled with joy.

I am confident.

I am at peace with

where I am in life.

I am worthy of a life

filled with fulfillment

and purpose.

I am in control of my

mind.

I am capable of overcoming any obstacle.

I am deserving of a life filled with peace and happiness.

I am surrounded by

positive people who

support me.

I am worthy of success and prosperity.

I am at peace with

myself and the world

around me.

I have a happy and fulfilling life.

I choose to focus on the good in every situation.

I choose to live each day
with joy and positivity.

I am worthy of a life

filled with success.

I am surrounded by positive, supportive people.

I am at peace with the present moment.

I am deserving of a life filled with love and fulfillment.

I choose to focus on my goals and aspirations.

I am capable of finding solutions to any problem.

I am at peace with the

journey of life.

I am grateful for my

many blessings.

I am in control of my thoughts and emotions.

I am surrounded by positive energy and love.

I am grateful for the

present moment and all

that it brings.

I am worthy of an

abundant life.

I am able to find joy and happiness in every situation.

I trust in my own
abilities and decisions.

I am deserving of a life filled with love, peace, and happiness.

I am strong and
accomplished.

I am grateful for my journey and all that I have learned.

I am capable of

managing my thoughts

and emotions.

I am in control of my reactions to stressful situations.

I am strong and capable

of facing any challenge.

I am worthy of love,

peace, and happiness.

I am deserving of a life filled with success and abundance.

I focus on my own progress, not perfection.

I am surrounded by a supportive network of friends and family.

I am grateful for the
opportunities life
presents to me.

I am deserving of a life filled with love and positivity.

I am strong and capable of overcoming any barrier.

I am at peace with my

past and excited for my

future.

I am deserving of a fulfilling and meaningful life.

I focus on the present
and let go of worries.

I am worthy of love and

happiness in all areas of

my life.

I am capable of finding
joy in even the most
difficult situations.

I am surrounded by positive energy and positivity.

I am deserving of

success and abundance

in all areas of my life.

I am capable of facing

any challenge.

I am grateful for my
health and well-being.

I am calm and centered

in every moment.

I am without worry.

I am capable of handling any situation with ease.

I am overcoming anxiety.

I am surrounded by love

and positivity.

I am strong and
resilient in the face of
stress.

I am letting go of the

past and future.

I am worthy of love and

happiness.

I trust my life's journey.

I am fearless.

I am enough just as I am.

I am surrounded by

abundance and

prosperity.

I am confident in my decisions and trust my intuition.

I am worthy of a life free

from anxiety.

I am grateful for the

peace and serenity in

my life.

I am capable of achieving my goals and dreams.

I am strong and capable
of handling anything
that comes my way.

I am at peace with the

uncertainty of life.

I am filled with love and

positivity.

I am joyful and

peaceful.

I am free from worry

and stress.

I am graceful and

resilient.

I am deserving of a life
filled with happiness
and success.

I am surrounded by a supportive network of people who love and care for me.

I am grateful for my life.

I am valid in my feelings.

I am under no threat

from the world.

I am calmer and more relaxed with each new day.

I am in control of my life.

Please Write A Review

Hello there!

Are you someone who believes in the power of positive affirmations and wants to experience greater fulfillment in life? If yes, then I have a question - how often do you find yourself scrolling through online stores or apps, searching for the perfect book that will help you deal with your anxiety? And when you finally find that book, how do you know if it's worth your time and money? Well, the answer is simple - you look for reviews from other readers who have already read the book!

This is where I need your help - I'm requesting you to leave an honest review of "101 Affirmations for Anxiety" to help others who are searching for a book that can help them cope with their anxiety. By leaving a review, you can provide an opportunity for someone else to experience the same positive impact that you experienced during your reading or listening experience.

Reviews are crucial for any author or book because they help potential readers decide if the book is the right fit for them. Your review can help someone who is struggling with anxiety find the support and guidance they need to overcome their fears and live an abundant life.

So, how can you leave a review? It's simple! You can go to the book's page on Amazon or Goodreads and leave your thoughts about the book. You can mention what you liked about the book, how it helped you, and who you would recommend it to. Your review can be short or long, as long as it's honest and from the heart.

Leaving a review can have a positive impact not just on potential readers but also on the author. Your feedback can help the author improve their work and create better content in the future. You can be a part of the author's journey and help them achieve their dreams.

Thank you for considering my request. Let's help others find the support and guidance they need to live a happier, more abundant life.

References

Do Positive Affirmations Work? What Experts Say. (2021, December 7). Cleveland Clinic Health Essentials. Retrieved February 1, 2023, from https://health.clevelandclinic.org/do-positive-affirmations-work/

Moore, C., & Nash, J. (2019, March 4). *Positive Daily Affirmations: Is There Science Behind It?* PositivePsychology.com. Retrieved February 1, 2023, from https://positivepsychology.com/daily-affirmations/

NIMH » Anxiety Disorders. (n.d.). NIMH. Retrieved February 2, 2023, from https://www.nimh.nih.gov/health/topics/anxiety-disorders

Using Affirmations - Harnessing Positive Thinking. (n.d.). Mind Tools. Retrieved February 1, 2023, from https://www.mindtools.com/air49f4/using-affirmations

www.ingramcontent.com/pod-product-compliance
Lightning Source LLC
Chambersburg PA
CBHW070825250726

48662CB00003B/1086